KATE ROSE

Holistic Momma Remedies

To my two incredible sons, Davey and Jordan,
Your curiosity and boundless imagination are the light that guides
my way. This book is a testament to the joy and wonder you bring
into my life each day. May you always chase your dreams with the
same passion and courage that you inspire in me.
With all my love and pride,
Mom

Contents

Introduction

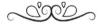

Motherhood is a journey of profound transformation and discovery. From the moment a woman learns she is expecting, her life becomes a tapestry of new experiences, emotions, and responsibilities. This transition, while joyous, also brings unique challenges, particularly in maintaining personal well-being while nurturing a new life. In an era where conventional medicine often focuses primarily on addressing symptoms and managing diseases, many mothers are turning to holistic remedies to complement their healthcare approach.

Purpose of the Book

This book, Holistic Momma Remedies, aims to provide a detailed exploration of holistic practices that can support mothers through the various stages of motherhood. Our goal is to offer practical, accessible information that goes beyond common knowledge, integrating time-honored wisdom with contemporary understanding to enrich your journey through pregnancy, postpartum recovery, and beyond.

Holistic health encompasses a broad spectrum of practices, from nutrition and natural remedies to mental and emotional wellness. It is an approach that considers the whole person—

body, mind, and spirit—rather than focusing solely on isolated symptoms. By adopting holistic remedies, mothers can address not only the physical changes and challenges they face but also nurture their emotional and mental health in a balanced and integrated way.

Why Holistic Remedies?

In a world where the pace of life is accelerating and the demands on mothers are increasing, holistic remedies offer a refreshing and compassionate alternative to conventional methods. They emphasize prevention, balance, and the body's natural ability to heal. Holistic practices often focus on self-care, natural treatments, and lifestyle adjustments that align with the body's inherent rhythms and needs.

For many mothers, holistic remedies provide a sense of empowerment and control over their health and well-being. These practices can complement conventional treatments, offering additional support in managing common pregnancy discomforts, supporting postpartum recovery, and fostering a nurturing environment for their growing families. By understanding and integrating holistic practices, mothers can create a more harmonious and supportive experience for themselves and their loved ones.

The Modern Mother's Journey

Today's mothers face a unique set of challenges. Balancing career, family life, and personal health can be overwhelming. Amidst these pressures, holistic remedies offer a pathway to achieving greater balance and well-being. This book will explore how holistic practices can help manage stress, enhance physical health, and foster emotional resilience.

The journey of motherhood is deeply personal, and there is no single path to achieving well-being. By exploring holistic remedies, we provide mothers with a range of tools and insights that can be tailored to their individual needs and circumstances. This guide will offer practical advice, backed by both traditional knowledge and contemporary research, to support mothers in making informed choices about their health.

What to Expect in This Book

Throughout this book, we will cover a variety of topics essential to holistic health and motherhood:

- **Chapter 1: The Foundations of Holistic Health** will provide an overview of the principles underlying holistic practices, including their historical context, core concepts, and scientific support.

- **Chapter 2: Nutrition and Diet for Motherhood** will delve into the importance of a balanced diet, offering customized dietary advice for pregnancy, postpartum recovery, and breastfeeding, as well as tips for managing common dietary issues.

- **Chapter 3: Natural Remedies for Common Pregnancy Discomforts** will explore practical solutions for managing pregnancy-related issues such as morning sickness, back pain, and stress through natural and non-pharmacological methods.

- **Chapter 4: Postpartum Recovery and Well-being** will focus on holistic approaches to physical and emotional recovery after childbirth, including strategies for managing postpartum depression and supporting breastfeeding.

- **Chapter 5: Infant Care through Holistic Lenses** will discuss holistic practices for caring for a newborn, including nutrition, sleep routines, and natural remedies for common infant ailments.

- **Chapter 6: Holistic Parenting Practices** will examine how to create a holistic home environment, support emotional

3

development, and build strong family bonds.

- **Chapter 7: Integrating Holistic Practices with Conventional Medicine** will address how to effectively combine holistic and conventional approaches, including real-life case studies and practical advice.

- **Chapter 8: Continuing Your Holistic Journey** will provide resources for ongoing education and personal growth, encouraging mothers to continue exploring and integrating holistic practices into their lives.

A Journey of Empowerment

As you embark on this journey through the pages of this book, we invite you to approach it with an open mind and a spirit of exploration. Holistic remedies offer a wealth of opportunities to enhance your health and well-being in a nurturing and integrated manner. By embracing these practices, you can empower yourself to navigate the challenges of motherhood with greater ease, balance, and fulfillment.

We hope that this guide will serve as a valuable resource, providing you with the knowledge and tools to support yourself and your family on this transformative journey. Welcome to a holistic approach to motherhood—one that honors the interconnectedness of body, mind, and spirit, and supports you every step of the way.

Chapter 1: The Foundations of Holistic Health

~~~
◦ᔆᑦᕐᔆ◦
~~~

1.1 Historical Context

Holistic health, a term that reflects an integrated approach to wellness, has deep roots in human history. Ancient civilizations, including those of China, India, and Greece, embraced holistic concepts long before they became popular in modern times. For instance, Traditional Chinese Medicine (TCM) dates back over 2,000 years and emphasizes the balance of Qi (life force energy) within the body. Similarly, Ayurvedic medicine, originating in India, promotes harmony through diet, lifestyle, and herbal treatments.

In ancient Greece, Hippocrates, often referred to as the father of medicine, advocated for treating the whole person rather than just symptoms. His approach emphasized the body's innate ability to heal itself and the importance of a balanced lifestyle. These historical practices laid the groundwork for

5

what we now understand as holistic health. The evolution of holistic health through the centuries reflects humanity's ongoing quest for a balanced and comprehensive approach to well-being. As modern medicine advanced, focusing on specific diseases and treatments, the holistic view remained a cornerstone in various traditional practices, serving as a reminder of the interconnections of the body, mind, and environment.

1.2 Core Principles of Holistic Health

At its heart, holistic health is built upon several core principles that set it apart from conventional medicine:

- Mind-Body Connection: Holistic health recognizes that mental and emotional states are deeply interconnected with physical health. Stress, for example, can manifest as physical ailments, while emotional well-being can significantly impact physical health. This principle underscores the importance of addressing psychological factors alongside physical symptoms.

- Balance and Harmony: A central tenet of holistic health is achieving balance and harmony within the body and with the external environment. This involves not only balancing physical needs but also ensuring emotional, spiritual, and social well-being. Practices such as yoga, meditation, and mindfulness are often employed to cultivate this balance.

- Personalized Care: Holistic health approaches are highly individualized. Rather than applying a one-size-fits-all treatment, holistic practitioners consider a person's unique physical, emotional, and environmental factors. This personalized approach allows for tailored treatments that address the root causes of health issues rather than just the symptoms.

- Prevention and Wellness: Holistic health places a strong emphasis on prevention and maintaining wellness rather than merely treating illness. This involves proactive measures such as healthy eating, regular exercise, and stress management to prevent health issues from arising in the first place.

1.3 The Science Behind Holistic Remedies

While holistic health often draws from traditional practices, modern scientific research has begun to validate many of its principles. For example:

- Mindfulness and Stress Reduction: Studies have shown that mindfulness practices, such as meditation and yoga, can reduce stress, lower blood pressure, and improve overall well-being. These findings support the holistic belief in the mind-body connection and the benefits of mental practices for physical health.

- Nutritional Science: The benefits of a balanced diet rich in whole foods, as emphasized in holistic nutrition, are well-documented. Research has confirmed that whole foods, such as fruits, vegetables, and whole grains, contribute to better health outcomes compared to processed foods.

- Herbal Medicine: Many traditional herbal remedies have been the subject of scientific studies that validate their efficacy. For example, ginger has been found to alleviate nausea, and chamomile has been shown to promote relaxation and improve sleep.

However, it's important to acknowledge that while many holistic remedies are supported by research, there are limitations and areas where evidence is still emerging. Holistic health practitioners must navigate the balance between traditional wisdom and scientific validation, ensuring that treatments are both effective and safe.

1.4 Integrating Holistic Health into Modern Life

Incorporating holistic health principles into modern life

requires an understanding of both traditional practices and contemporary advancements. This integration can be challenging, particularly as conventional medicine often focuses on treating symptoms rather than promoting overall well-being. Modern mothers, in particular, may find holistic approaches beneficial as they navigate the complex demands of motherhood.

Holistic remedies offer ways to manage stress, improve physical health, and support emotional well-being, which can be especially valuable during the trans formative journey of motherhood.

By blending time-tested practices with current research, mothers can create a personalized approach to health that supports not only their own well-being but also the health of their families. Embracing holistic health is about more than just adopting new remedies; it's about cultivating a lifestyle that values balance, prevention, and comprehensive care.

Chapter 2: Nutrition and Diet for Motherhood

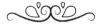

2.1 Holistic Nutrition Basics

Nutrition forms the bedrock of holistic health, with a focus on whole, unprocessed foods that support overall well-being. For mothers, whether pregnant, postpartum, or breastfeeding, nutritional needs are particularly crucial. Holistic nutrition emphasizes not just what you eat but how your diet interacts with your body's natural processes and environment.

Whole Foods Approach

- Definition and Benefits: Whole foods are foods that are minimally processed and free from artificial additives. These include fruits, vegetables, whole grains, nuts, seeds, and lean proteins. The benefits of a whole foods diet are manifold: it supports optimal digestion, provides essential nutrients, and helps maintain a balanced blood sugar level. For mothers, this translates to better energy levels, improved mood stability, and overall enhanced health.

- Nutrient Density: Holistic nutrition stresses the importance of nutrient-dense foods, which provide a high amount of vitamins, minerals, and other beneficial compounds relative to their calorie content. Nutrient-dense choices, such as leafy greens, berries, and fatty fish, support maternal and infant health.

- Food Synergy: The concept of food synergy refers to the idea that nutrients in whole foods work together to enhance health benefits. For example, the vitamin C in citrus fruits can improve the absorption of iron from plant-based sources like spinach. Holistic nutrition encourages combining foods to maximize their health benefits.

2.2 Customized Diet Plans

The dietary needs of mothers vary depending on their stage in motherhood. A holistic approach involves customizing nutrition plans to meet these specific needs.

Pregnancy

-Essential Nutrients: During pregnancy, key nutrients include folate, iron, calcium, and omega-3 fatty acids. Folate supports fetal neural development, iron is crucial for blood production, calcium strengthens bones, and omega-3s support brain development. Sources include leafy greens, fortified cereals, dairy products, and fatty fish.

- Managing Common Issues: Pregnancy can bring about issues such as morning sickness and food cravings. Holistic remedies include ginger tea for nausea and small, frequent meals to manage hunger and prevent nausea. Incorporating nutrient-dense snacks can also help address cravings healthily.

Postpartum

- Recovery and Healing: After childbirth, the body requires nutrients to recover and support healing. High-protein foods, such as lean meats, especially organ meats and legumes, are beneficial for tissue repair. Foods rich in vitamins C and E, like citrus fruits and nuts, aid in skin healing and overall recovery. - Energy and Mood Support: Postpartum mothers often experience fatigue and mood swings. Complex carbohydrates, such as oats and sweet potatoes, provide sustained energy, while foods rich in omega-3 fatty acids, like walnuts and flax seeds, support emotional balance. Mothers are encapsulating their placenta after birth to make capsules to help replenish nutrients for the sake of more energy and mood support.

Breastfeeding

- Nutritional Support for Milk Production: Breastfeeding mothers need additional calories and nutrients to support milk production. Adequate hydration is also crucial. Foods that support lactation include oats, fennel seeds, and garlic. A balanced diet with a variety of nutrients ensures both mother and baby receive essential vitamins and minerals. Drinks like coconut water added with fresh fruit juice and salt make a great hydration cocktail and help aid in milk production.

- Monitoring Allergies and Sensitivities: As breastfeeding mothers introduce foods into their diet, it's important to monitor for potential allergens or sensitivities in the baby. Keeping a food diary can help identify any correlations between the mother's diet and the baby's reactions.

2.3 Managing Common Dietary Issues

Food Sensitivities and Allergies

- Identifying Triggers: Food sensitivities and allergies can affect both the mother and baby. Common culprits include dairy, gluten, and nuts. Holistic approaches involve an elimination diet to identify triggers, followed by reintroducing foods to pinpoint the problem areas.

- Alternative Options: For those with sensitivities, alternative foods are available. Almond or oat milk can replace dairy, while gluten-free grains like quinoa and rice can substitute for wheat. It's important to ensure that these alternatives still provide necessary nutrients.

Cravings and Overeating

- Healthy Craving Management: Cravings during pregnancy and postpartum can be managed with healthier alternatives. For example, if craving sweets, opt for fruit or dark chocolate rather than sugary snacks. Ensuring balanced meals and snacks can help curb excessive cravings.

- Mindful Eating: Practicing mindful eating—being aware of what and how much you eat—can help manage portion sizes and prevent overeating. Techniques include eating slowly, savoring each bite, and paying attention to hunger cues.

Dietary Deficiencies

- Common Deficiencies: Nutrient deficiencies, such as low iron or vitamin D, can impact health. Holistic approaches involve incorporating foods rich in these nutrients and considering supplements if necessary. For instance, incorporating iron-rich foods like lentils and spinach can help prevent anemia.

- Testing and Monitoring: Regular check-ups and nutritional testing can help monitor deficiencies and adjust dietary plans accordingly. A holistic nutritionist or healthcare provider can offer personalized advice based on individual needs.

2.4 Practical Meal Planning Tips

Creating Balanced Meals

-Meal Structure: Aim for balanced meals that include a variety of food groups: vegetables, proteins, healthy fats, and whole grains. A typical plate might include a serving of grilled salmon (protein and omega-3s), quinoa (whole grain), and a side of roasted vegetables (vitamins and minerals). -Meal Prep Strategies: Preparing meals in advance can simplify healthy eating. Batch cooking and storing meals in portion-sized containers can make it easier to adhere to a balanced diet. Making freezer-friendly dishes to use in the future can help when you know your schedule will change. Incorporating a variety of recipes and seasonal ingredients can keep meals interesting and nutritious.

Incorporating Holistic Foods
- Super-foods and Herbs: Adding super-foods like chia seeds, spirulina, and turmeric to your diet can provide additional health benefits. These foods are known for their high nutrient content and potential health-boosting properties.
- Herbal Teas and Supplements: Herbal teas such as peppermint or chamomile can support digestion and relaxation. Supplements like papaya enzymes can aid in gut health, which is integral to overall well-being. Prenatal multivitamins are good to take well into postpartum and all the way to the end of your breastfeeding journey. Also, a good source of fish oil in combination with a prenatal will ensure a balanced vitamin and mineral intake.

Family-Friendly Recipes
- Nutrient-Dense Recipes: Create meals that are both nutritious and appealing to the whole family. Recipes like veggie-loaded soups baked sweet potatoes with beans, and fruit smoothies with hidden veggies, chia seeds, and protein can provide essential nutrients while catering to varied tastes. If your kids are anything like mine, I load veggies (zucchini and squash are the easiest to mask) into anything and everything possible.
- Involving Family: Engaging family members in meal

planning and preparation can make healthy eating a shared goal. Involving children in cooking can also teach them about nutrition and encourage healthy eating habits.

Chapter 3: Natural Remedies for Common Pregnancy Discomforts

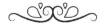

Pregnancy is a beautiful yet complex journey that can bring about a range of physical and emotional challenges. While modern medicine provides many solutions, natural remedies offer additional ways to manage common pregnancy discomforts. This chapter explores a variety of holistic approaches to alleviate issues such as morning sickness, back pain, and mental stress, providing safe and effective options to support a healthy pregnancy.

3.1 Morning Sickness

Morning sickness, characterized by nausea and vomiting, affects many pregnant women, especially during the first trimester. While it is commonly referred to as "morning" sickness, it can occur at any time of day. Natural remedies can help ease these symptoms and support overall well-being.

- Ginger: Ginger is a well-known remedy for nausea. It can be consumed in various forms, including ginger tea, ginger ale (with real ginger), or ginger candies. Research suggests that ginger helps to reduce nausea and vomiting by influencing gastrointestinal motility.

- Peppermint: Peppermint is another effective remedy for nausea. Peppermint tea or sucking on peppermint lozenges can help calm the stomach. The menthol in peppermint has soothing properties that may help relieve nausea.

- Acupressure: Acupressure, a technique that involves applying pressure to specific points on the body, can help alleviate nausea. The P6 point, located on the inner wrist, is particularly effective. Wristbands designed for acupressure, such as sea bands, are available and can be worn throughout the day.

- Small, Frequent Meals: Eating small, frequent meals can help stabilize blood sugar levels and reduce nausea. Opt for bland, easy-to-digest foods like crackers, toast, and bananas. Avoiding large, rich meals can prevent overwhelming the digestive system.

3.2 Back Pain and Body Aches

As pregnancy progresses, the growing baby and changes in body mechanics can lead to back pain and general body aches. Several natural approaches can help alleviate these discomforts:

- Prenatal Yoga: Prenatal yoga is a gentle exercise that helps strengthen the muscles supporting the back and pelvis. Poses such as cat-cow, child's pose, and pelvic tilts can improve flexibility and reduce pain. Always consult with a healthcare provider before starting any new exercise regimen.

- Prenatal Massage: Specialized prenatal massage can relieve muscle tension and improve circulation. Look for a certified massage therapist experienced in prenatal care to ensure safety and effectiveness.

- Warm Compresses and Baths: Applying a warm compress

to the lower back or taking a warm bath can help relax tense muscles and ease discomfort. Avoid hot temperatures to ensure safety for both mother and baby.

- Proper Posture and Ergonomics: Maintaining good posture and using ergonomic support while sitting or standing can reduce back strain. Consider using a supportive chair with good lumbar support and be mindful of body mechanics when lifting objects.

3.3 Mental Wellness and Stress Management

Pregnancy can be a time of heightened emotions and stress. Managing mental wellness is crucial for both maternal and fetal health. Holistic approaches can help support emotional balance and stress relief.

- Mindfulness and Meditation: Mindfulness practices and meditation can reduce stress and promote relaxation. Techniques such as deep breathing, guided imagery, and progressive muscle relaxation can help calm the mind and alleviate anxiety.

- Supportive Relationships: Building a support network of friends, family, healthcare providers, birth coach, and or a doula can provide emotional support and practical assistance. Talking about your feelings and concerns with trusted individuals can help alleviate stress and provide reassurance.

- Journaling: Keeping a journal can be a therapeutic way to process emotions and reflect on your pregnancy experience. Writing about your thoughts, hopes, and concerns can provide a sense of clarity and emotional release.

- Adequate Rest and Sleep: Prioritizing rest and sleep is essential for managing stress and maintaining overall health. Creating a calming bedtime routine and ensuring a comfortable sleep environment can improve sleep quality.

3.4 Other Common Pregnancy Discomforts

In addition to morning sickness, back pain, and stress, there are other common pregnancy discomforts that natural remedies can address:

- Heartburn: Eating smaller meals, avoiding spicy and acidic foods, and drinking herbal teas like chamomile or ginger can help manage heartburn. Sleeping with the head elevated can also prevent acid re-flux during the night.

- Leg Cramps: To alleviate leg cramps, ensure adequate hydration and maintain a balanced intake of calcium and magnesium. Stretching the legs before bed and gently massaging the affected area can also help relieve cramps.

- Swelling: Mild swelling in the feet and ankles is common during pregnancy. Elevating the legs, staying hydrated, and wearing comfortable shoes can help manage swelling. Limiting salt intake can also reduce fluid retention.

3.5 Safe Use of Essential Oils

Essential oils can be a helpful addition to a holistic approach, offering benefits for various pregnancy-related symptoms. However, it's essential to use them safely and consult with a healthcare provider before use.

- Lavender: Lavender essential oil is known for its calming properties and can help with stress and sleep issues. Use it in a diffuser or dilute it with a carrier oil for topical application. Also can be used as a bug deterrent.

- Frankincense: Frankincense may help with anxiety and emotional well-being. It can be used in a diffuser or applied topically in a diluted form.

- Caution with Essential Oils: Not all essential oils are safe for use during pregnancy. Avoid oils that are considered potentially harmful, such as rosemary and sage, and consult with a professional aromatherapist for guidance.

Chapter 4: Postpartum Recovery and Well-being

The postpartum period, often referred to as the fourth trimester, is a critical phase in a mother's journey. This time of transition brings both physical and emotional changes as the body recovers from childbirth and adjusts to caring for a new baby. Holistic remedies offer valuable support during this period, helping mothers navigate recovery and maintain overall well-being. This chapter explores natural approaches to postpartum recovery, including physical healing, emotional support, and breastfeeding assistance.

4.1 Physical Recovery- Postpartum Healing

- Rest and Recovery: Adequate rest is crucial for physical healing after childbirth. The body has undergone significant changes and stress, and it needs time to recover. Prioritize sleep when possible, and accept help from family and friends to manage household responsibilities and care for the baby.

- Pelvic Floor Health: Strengthening the pelvic floor is

important for recovery and long-term health. Gentle pelvic floor exercises, such as Kegels, dead bug, and bird dogs can help restore muscle tone and support urinary and reproductive health. Consult a pelvic floor therapist for personalized guidance if needed. Chiropractic adjustments and massage are good for pelvic floor pain as well.

- Postpartum Pain Management: Common postpartum discomforts include perineal pain, after-pains, and abdominal soreness. Natural remedies such as sitz baths with Epsom salts or herbal infusions (e.g., witch hazel) can soothe and heal. Applying cold packs can also reduce inflammation and provide relief.

Nutrition for Recovery

- Nutrient-Rich Foods: A well-balanced diet supports postpartum recovery by providing essential nutrients for healing and energy. Focus on nutrient-dense foods such as lean proteins, whole grains, fruits, and vegetables. Iron-rich foods like leafy greens and legumes help replenish blood levels, while omega-3 fatty acids from fish and flax-seeds support overall recovery.

- Herbal Supplements: Certain herbs can aid in postpartum recovery. For example, red clover tea is thought to support hormonal balance, while ginger can help with digestion and reduce inflammation. Always consult a healthcare provider before using herbal supplements to ensure they are safe and appropriate.

4.2 Emotional Health

Postpartum Mood

- Understanding Postpartum Depression: Postpartum depression (PPD) is a serious condition affecting many new mothers, characterized by persistent sadness, anxiety, and mood swings. It is important to seek professional help if symptoms of PPD arise. Holistic approaches can complement conventional treatments but should not replace them.

- Emotional Support: Building a support network is essential for emotional well-being. Connect with family, friends, or support groups to share experiences and seek encouragement. Postpartum doulas and lactation consultants can also provide practical and emotional support.

- Mindfulness and Relaxation: Mindfulness techniques such as meditation, deep breathing, and progressive muscle relaxation can help manage stress and improve mood. Setting aside a few minutes each day for relaxation can provide a sense of calm and emotional balance.

Self-Care Practices

- Journaling: Writing about your experiences and emotions can be a therapeutic way to process the changes of motherhood. Journaling can help you reflect on your feelings and track your recovery progress.

- Gentle Exercise: Gradual, gentle exercise, such as walking or postnatal yoga, can improve mood, increase energy levels, and aid physical recovery. Always consult with a healthcare provider before starting any new exercise routine.

4.3 Breastfeeding Support
Nutrition for Lactation
- Supporting Milk Production: Adequate nutrition and hydration are key to maintaining a healthy milk supply. Foods such as oats, barley, and fenugreek seeds are believed to support lactation. Consuming a balanced diet rich in vitamins and minerals also benefits both mother and baby.

- Managing Common Issues: Common breastfeeding challenges include sore nipples, engorgement, and difficulty with latch. Applying lanolin cream to sore nipples, using warm compresses to ease engorgement, and seeking guidance from a lactation consultant can help address these issues.

- Lactation Teas: Herbal teas formulated for lactation, such as those containing fenugreek, blessed thistle, or fennel, are traditionally used to support milk production. These teas can be a soothing and supportive addition to your postpartum routine.

4.4 Addressing Common Postpartum Issues
Fatigue

- Managing Fatigue Postpartum fatigue is common due to disrupted sleep patterns and the demands of caring for a newborn. Establishing a consistent sleep routine, taking naps when possible, and accepting help with baby care can help manage fatigue.

- Nutritional Support: Consuming nutrient-rich snacks and meals throughout the day can provide sustained energy. Include snacks that combine protein and complex carbohydrates, such as yogurt with fruit or whole-grain crackers with nut butter.

Hair Loss

- Understanding Postpartum Hair Loss: Temporary hair loss is a common occurrence after childbirth due to hormonal changes. This condition is typically short-lived and resolves on its own. To support hair health, maintain a balanced diet and consider gentle hair care practices.

Constipation

- Digestive Health: Constipation can be an issue postpartum due to hormonal changes and dietary adjustments. Increasing fiber intake through fruits, vegetables, and whole grains, and drinking plenty of water, can help maintain regular bowel movements. Gentle physical activity, such as walking, can also support digestive health.

4.5 Building a Supportive Environment
Creating a Positive Atmosphere

- Home Environment: Create a calming and supportive home environment to facilitate postpartum recovery. Organize a comfortable and accessible space for feeding and bonding with the baby. Consider using soothing colors, soft lighting, and relaxing music to create a peaceful atmosphere.

- Family Involvement: Engage family members in supporting your postpartum journey. Open communication about your needs and expectations can help ensure that you receive the necessary assistance and understanding during this time.

Chapter 5: Infant Care through Holistic Lenses

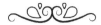

The early days of a newborn's life are a period of immense growth and adjustment for both the baby and the parents. Holistic infant care emphasizes nurturing the baby's physical, emotional, and developmental needs in a way that supports overall well-being. This chapter explores holistic approaches to infant care, including natural remedies for common issues, creating a nurturing environment, and fostering early development.

5.1 Nutrition and Feeding
Breastfeeding Support
- Nutritional Benefits: Breastfeeding provides optimal nutrition and supports the baby's immune system. It is also beneficial for the mother, promoting postpartum recovery and enhancing emotional bonding. Ensure a balanced diet for the mother to support milk production and quality.
Managing Challenges

Breastfeeding can present a range of challenges, particularly in the early days. Addressing these issues promptly and effectively is crucial to ensure a successful breastfeeding experience and to support both mother and baby.

-Latching Difficulties: A proper latch is essential for effective breastfeeding and preventing discomfort. If the baby is not latching correctly, it can lead to inadequate milk intake and sore nipples.

- Consult a Lactation Consultant: A lactation consultant can provide personalized guidance on achieving a proper latch. They can offer hands-on assistance, demonstrate techniques, and help resolve issues that might be hindering successful breastfeeding.

- Try Different Positions: Experiment with different breastfeeding positions to find the most comfortable and effective one for both mother and baby. Common positions include the cradle hold, football hold, and side-lying position. For clogged ducts try positioning the baby's nose in that duct's way to empty it, moving the baby around the breast. Each position can provide different benefits and may improve the latch.

Sore Nipples

Sore nipples are a common issue, especially in the initial weeks of breastfeeding. Proper care and prevention strategies can help alleviate discomfort.

- Use Natural Remedies: Applying coconut oil or expressed breast milk to sore nipples can provide soothing relief and promote healing. Both have natural antibacterial properties that can help prevent infection. Gently massage a small amount onto the nipples after feeding and allow it to air dry.

- Warm Compresses: Using warm compresses before breastfeeding can help with engorgement and improve milk flow, which may make latching easier and reduce discomfort. Soak a clean cloth in warm water, wring it out, and apply it to the breasts for a few minutes. Do this before each session to ensure an easy latch.

- Keep Nipples Dry: Use nipple pads to manage leaks and keep nipples dry between feedings. Moist environments can lead to cracked and bleeding nipples. Change pads frequently to ensure that the skin remains dry and protected.

Concerns About Milk Supply

Concerns about milk supply can be stressful and may affect the breastfeeding experience. It is essential to address these concerns with appropriate strategies and support.

- Frequent Nursing: Frequent nursing can help stimulate milk production. Aim to feed the baby on demand and ensure they are breastfeeding effectively. The more often the baby nurses, the more milk the body will produce.

- Hydration and Nutrition: Staying well-hydrated and maintaining a nutritious diet can support milk production. Foods such as oats, nuts, and leafy greens are believed to help enhance milk supply. Drink plenty of water and eat balanced meals to nourish both mother and baby.

- Consult Professionals: If concerns about milk supply persist, consult with a lactation consultant or healthcare provider. They can offer advice on techniques to increase supply and determine if any underlying issues need to be addressed. Many mothers face challenges during their breastfeeding journey, and seeking support is crucial. Don't hesitate to reach out to a lactation consultant for guidance. They can provide valuable support and address specific concerns, which can make a significant difference in overcoming breastfeeding challenges. Donor milk is also another viable option. Sometimes it has nothing to do with milk supply, some babies have tongue/lip ties or even a buccal tie that is causing the issues.

- Join Support Groups: Consider joining a breastfeeding support group where you can share experiences, gain advice, and find encouragement from other mothers. A good place to find a milk donor if needed. These groups can provide emotional support and practical tips for managing common issues.

Introducing Solid Foods

- Timing and Guidelines: Solid foods can typically be introduced around 4-6 months of age, when the baby shows signs of readiness, such as sitting up with support and showing interest in food. Start with single-ingredient purees and gradually introduce a variety of foods or look into baby-led weaning to start the eating process.

- Nutrient-Dense Choices: Focus on nutrient-dense foods that provide essential vitamins and minerals. Options include pureed vegetables (e.g., spinach, kale, green beans, sweet potatoes, carrots), fruits (e.g., blueberries, avocado, apples, pears), and iron-rich foods (e.g., pureed meats, lentils, oatmeal).

5.2 Sleep and Routines

Establishing Healthy Sleep Habits

- Creating a Sleep Environment: A calming sleep environment supports better sleep for both baby and parents. Co-sleeping has been proven to create independence, confidence, and self-reliance. It also encourages breastfeeding at night and can help babies sleep on their backs which could reduce the risk of SIDS. Ensure the baby's sleep area is safe, with a firm mattress and no loose bedding. Use soft, natural fabrics and maintain a comfortable room temperature. Sound machines can help with keeping the baby asleep.

- Sleep Routine: Establishing a consistent bedtime routine can help the baby differentiate between day and night. Activities such as a warm bath, gentle massage, and quiet lullabies can signal that it's time for sleep. Consistency is key to creating a sense of security and routine.

5.3 Soothing Techniques
Natural Remedies for Common Issues
- Colic and Gas: Colic and gas can cause discomfort for infants. Gentle tummy massage, bicycle legs, warm baths, and chiropractic adjustments can help relieve gas. A pacifier can also provide comfort and help with self-soothing. Pro and Prebiotic drops as well as vitamin D drops help too.
- Teething: Teething can be uncomfortable for babies. Offer teething toys that are safe for chewing. Chilling a teething ring or offering cold, clean washcloths with expressed breast milk to chew on can soothe sore gums. A gentle massage with your finger can help the tooth come through the gums and ease pain. Avoid teething gels or medications without consulting a pediatrician. Use homeopathic liquid pouches as an alternative(e.g. Camilia)

5.4 Bonding and Emotional Development
Building Strong Emotional Connections
- Skin-to-Skin Contact: Skin-to-skin contact immediately after birth and during the early days fosters bonding and helps regulate the baby's body temperature, heart rate, and stress levels. This contact also supports breastfeeding and emotional connection.
- Responsive Care-giving: Pay attention to the baby's cues and respond promptly to their needs. This approach builds trust and helps the baby feel secure and understood. Gentle and consistent responses to crying, feeding, and sleep needs

promote emotional well-being.

- Early Interaction: Engage with the baby through talking, singing, and reading. Eye contact, gentle touch, and verbal communication support language development and emotional bonding.

5.5 Creating a Holistic Environment
Natural and Safe Products

- Choosing Non-Toxic Products: Select non-toxic, hypoallergenic products to minimize exposure to harmful chemicals. Read the labels and research the company to see if the brand can be trusted. Opt for organic cotton clothing, natural cleaning products, and chemical-free skincare items.

- Eco-Friendly Practices: Incorporate Eco-friendly practices into infant care, such as using cloth diapers or biodegradable options, and choosing sustainable toys and products. This approach supports environmental well-being and reduces exposure to potentially harmful substances.

Encouraging Development

- Sensory Stimulation: Provide a variety of sensory experiences to support the baby's development. Activities such as playing with textured toys, listening to different sounds, and exploring safe, colorful objects can stimulate sensory and cognitive development.

- Physical Activity: Encourage physical activity through tummy time and safe, supervised play. Tummy time helps strengthen the baby's neck and upper body muscles, promoting motor development and coordination.

5.6 Addressing Common Concerns
Dealing with Common Illnesses

Fever and Illness: When your baby has a fever or is unwell, closely monitor their symptoms and seek guidance from a pediatrician for appropriate treatment. It's often beneficial to allow the fever to run its natural course as this helps the body fight off infection. Ensure that your baby stays well-hydrated. If the fever reaches 105 degrees Fahrenheit, you should give the baby a lukewarm bath—avoid water that is too hot or too cold to prevent discomfort. Additionally, using a humidifier can help ease breathing and provide comfort.

- Skin Care: Baby's skin is delicate and may be prone to issues like diaper rash or eczema. Use natural, fragrance-free products for skincare and ensure frequent diaper changes to prevent irritation. Applying a barrier cream or coconut oil can soothe and protect sensitive skin.

Chapter 6: Holistic Approaches to Parenting

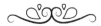

Parenting is a profound journey that involves nurturing, guiding, and supporting a child's development. Holistic parenting goes beyond traditional methods to encompass the emotional, physical, and spiritual well-being of both the child and the parent. This chapter explores holistic parenting practices, including creating a balanced family environment, fostering emotional intelligence, and integrating mindful parenting techniques.

6.1 Creating a Balanced Family Environment
Nurturing a Positive Atmosphere

- Open Communication: Foster a family environment where open and honest communication is encouraged. Encourage family members to express their thoughts and feelings and actively listen to each other. This practice builds trust and strengthens relationships.

- Quality Time Together: Spend quality time together as

a family to build strong bonds and create lasting memories. Engage in activities that everyone enjoys, such as family meals, outdoor adventures, or game nights. Prioritize meaningful interactions to strengthen family connections.

- Creating a Safe Space: Ensure that your home is a safe and supportive environment. Designate areas for relaxation, play, and study, and maintain a clutter-free, organized space to promote a sense of calm and order.

Promoting Healthy Family Dynamics

- Setting Boundaries: Establishing clear boundaries helps create a structured environment where everyone knows what to expect. Set consistent rules and routines while allowing flexibility for individual needs and preferences.

- Encouraging Independence: Support your child's growing independence by allowing them to make age-appropriate choices and learn from their experiences. Encourage problem-solving and decision-making skills while providing guidance and support.

- Modeling Positive Behavior: Children often learn by observing their parents. Model positive behaviors such as empathy, respect, and resilience. Demonstrating these traits can teach your child how to navigate relationships and handle challenges effectively.

6.2 Fostering Emotional Intelligence
Understanding and Managing Emotions
- Emotion Coaching: Help your child understand and manage their emotions by providing validation and support. Acknowledge their feelings and guide them in expressing and coping with emotions in a healthy way.

- Teaching Empathy: Encourage empathy by discussing different perspectives and practicing kindness. Use stories, role-playing, and real-life situations to teach your child how to understand and respond to the emotions of others.

- Modeling Emotional Regulation: Demonstrate effective emotional regulation by managing your own emotions calmly and constructively. Show how to handle stress and setbacks in a balanced manner, which helps your child learn similar skills.

Building Resilience

- Encouraging Problem-Solving: Support your child's development of resilience by allowing them to face challenges and solve problems independently. Provide guidance and encouragement while allowing them to experience the natural consequences of their actions.

- Celebrating Efforts: Acknowledge and celebrate your child's efforts and achievements, regardless of the outcome. Emphasize the value of perseverance and hard work, which fosters a growth mindset and resilience.

6.3 Integrating Mindful Parenting Techniques
Mindfulness Practices

- Being Present: Practice being fully present during interactions with your child. Engage in activities with attention and intention, minimizing distractions such as phones or multitasking. Being present strengthens your connection and enhances communication.

- Mindful Listening: Practice active and mindful listening when your child is speaking. Give them your full attention, maintain eye contact, and respond thoughtfully. This practice fosters a deeper understanding and respect in the parent-child relationship.

- Mindful Responses: Pause and reflect before responding to challenging behaviors or situations. Mindful responses allow you to address issues calmly and thoughtfully, avoiding reactive or impulsive reactions.

Incorporating Mindfulness into Daily Routines

- Mindful Activities: Integrate mindfulness into daily routines by incorporating activities such as mindful eating, breathing exercises, or gratitude practices. Encourage your child to participate in these activities to develop their own mindfulness skills.

- Family Mindfulness Practices: Engage in family mindfulness practices such as meditation or yoga. These activities promote relaxation, reduce stress, and create a sense of unity within the family.

6.4 Holistic Discipline Approaches
Positive Discipline Techniques

- Guidance over Punishment: Focus on guiding rather than punishing. Use techniques such as natural consequences, problem-solving discussions, and setting clear expectations to address misbehavior. Positive discipline encourages learning and growth.

- Consistency and Fairness: Be consistent and fair in applying discipline. Clearly communicate expectations and consequences, and ensure that rules are applied equally to all family members. Consistency helps build trust and understanding.

- Empowering Choices: Provide choices and involve your child in decision-making processes. Allowing them to make choices within set boundaries promotes responsibility and independence.

Encouraging Self-Reflection

- Reflective Conversations: Engage in reflective conversations with your child about their behavior and emotions. Discuss what went well, what could be improved, and how they can approach similar situations differently in the future.

- Modeling Self-Reflection: Demonstrate self-reflection by discussing your own experiences and learning from mistakes. Modeling this behavior helps your child understand the value of reflection and continuous improvement.

6.5 Supporting Development Through Play and Learning

Play as a Learning Tool

- Educational Play: Incorporate educational play into your child's daily routine. Provide toys and activities that stimulate creativity, problem-solving, and critical thinking. Activities such as building blocks, puzzles, and art projects support cognitive development.

- Interactive Learning: Engage in interactive learning experiences such as reading together, exploring nature, and participating in hands-on activities. These experiences foster curiosity and a love for learning.

- Safe Exploration: Create opportunities for safe exploration and discovery. Allow your child to explore their environment, try new activities, and pursue their interests. Support their curiosity and provide guidance as needed.

- Fostering Creativity: Encourage creative expression through various mediums such as drawing, music, and storytelling. Creative activities promote emotional expression and cognitive development.

Chapter 7: Holistic Approaches to Family Wellness

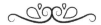

Family wellness encompasses the overall health and harmony of the household, integrating physical, emotional, and spiritual well-being for each family member. Adopting holistic approaches can enhance family life, improve relationships, and promote a balanced and fulfilling environment. This chapter explores strategies for maintaining family wellness, including natural health practices, effective communication, and creating a supportive home environment.

7.1 Natural Health Practices
Nutrition and Diet

- Whole Foods Approach: Emphasize a diet rich in whole, unprocessed foods to support overall health. Incorporate plenty of fruits, vegetables, whole grains, lean proteins, and healthy fats. A balanced diet contributes to physical well-being and energy levels for all family members.

- Meal Planning and Preparation: Plan and prepare meals

together as a family to encourage healthy eating habits. Involve children in age-appropriate cooking tasks to teach them about nutrition and foster a positive relationship with food.

- Mindful Eating: Practice mindful eating by focusing on the sensory experience of eating. Encourage family members to eat slowly, savor their food, and listen to their body's hunger and fullness cues.

Physical Activity

- Family Exercise: Incorporate physical activity into family routines through enjoyable activities. Engage in activities such as hiking, biking, dancing, or playing sports together. Regular exercise promotes physical health, strengthens bonds, and reduces stress.

- Active Lifestyle: Encourage an active lifestyle by integrating movement into daily routines. Opt for walking or biking instead of driving short distances, and encourage playtime that involves physical activity.

- Setting Goals: Set collective fitness goals and track progress as a family. Celebrate achievements and milestones to maintain motivation and create a sense of accomplishment.

Natural Health Remedies

Herbal Supplements: Explore a variety of herbal supplements and remedies that can support overall family wellness. For example:

- Echinacea: Known for its potential to enhance immune health, echinacea may help prevent or shorten the duration of colds and infections.

- Chamomile: Often used to promote relaxation and alleviate anxiety, chamomile can also aid in digestive comfort and improve sleep quality.

- Ginger: Ginger is commonly used to support digestive

health, reduce nausea, and ease muscle pain and inflammation.

- Turmeric: With its anti-inflammatory properties, turmeric can support joint health and may help with conditions such as arthritis.

- Peppermint: Peppermint can relieve digestive issues like bloating and gas, and its cooling properties may help alleviate headaches and muscle pain.

- Lavender: Lavender is known for its calming effects and can be used to promote relaxation, reduce stress, and improve sleep quality, as well as bug repellent.

- Elderberry: Elderberry is often used to support the immune system and may help reduce the severity and duration of cold and flu symptoms.

-Eucalyptus: Eucalyptus can support respiratory health. Incorporate essential oils through diffusers, topical applications (diluted with carrier oils), or bath soaks.

7.2 Effective Communication
Open and Honest Dialogue

- Encouraging Expression: Create an environment where family members feel comfortable expressing their thoughts and feelings. Encourage open dialogue by actively listening and validating each person's perspective.

- Conflict Resolution: Address conflicts and disagreements with empathy and problem-solving skills. Approach conflicts with a focus on understanding and finding mutually acceptable solutions. Avoid blame and criticism in favor of constructive communication.

- Family Meetings: Hold regular family meetings to discuss important matters, share updates, and address any issues. Use these meetings as a platform for collaborative decision-making and to strengthen family connections.

- Emotional Check-Ins: Regularly check in with each family member to assess their emotional well-being. Offer support and encouragement, and provide a safe space for discussing feelings and concerns.

- Building Resilience: Support each family member's emotional resilience by fostering a positive mindset and coping skills. Encourage self-care practices and stress management techniques, such as mindfulness and relaxation exercises.

- Bonding Activities: Prioritize quality time together by engaging in activities that strengthen relationships. Activities such as family game nights, shared hobbies, or outings promote bonding and create meaningful experiences.

- Unstructured Time: Allow for unstructured, spontaneous time together. This can include casual conversations, impromptu outings, or simply relaxing and enjoying each other's company.

7.3 Creating a Supportive Home Environment
Comfort and Safety

- Creating a Sanctuary: Design your home to be a comfortable and nurturing space. Use calming colors, natural materials, and cozy furnishings to create a soothing atmosphere. Ensure that each family member has a personal space where they can relax and recharge.

- Safety Measures: Implement safety measures to protect all family members. Childproof the home, maintain smoke detectors, and ensure that emergency supplies are readily available. A safe environment fosters peace of mind and security.

Organizational Harmony

- Decluttering: Maintain an organized and clutter-free home to promote a sense of calm and order. Regularly declutter and organize spaces to reduce stress and improve functionality.

- Household Routines: Establish household routines to create structure and predictability. This can include daily chores, meal times, and bedtime routines. Consistent routines support family harmony and reduce the likelihood of conflicts.

Spiritual Well-being

Explore and integrate your family's values and spiritual beliefs into daily life by engaging in practices that resonate with those principles, such as gratitude rituals, community service, or spiritual reflection. Incorporate mindfulness practices to enhance family wellness by fostering moments of reflection, meditation, or prayer, which can cultivate a sense of inner peace and deepen your family's connection.

7.4 Balancing Work and Family Life
Time Management

Prioritizing: Effectively manage your time by prioritizing family activities and responsibilities. For instance, if you set clear goals such as dedicating time for family dinners, work projects, and personal self-care, you can create a balanced schedule that ensures each area receives attention. For example, you might allocate evenings for family dinners and quality time, reserve certain hours during the workday for focused tasks, and set aside weekends for personal hobbies or relaxation.

Flexible Scheduling: Be adaptable with your schedule to meet evolving family needs. For instance, if an unexpected event comes up, such as a child's school performance or a last-minute work deadline, adjust your plans to accommodate these changes while still maintaining family time. Flexibility allows you to embrace spontaneous activities and ensures that family connections remain a priority, even when plans need to shift.

Self-Care for Parents

- Personal Well-being: Prioritize self-care to maintain physical and emotional health. Engage in activities that rejuvenate and relax you, such as exercise, hobbies, or socializing with friends.

- Support Networks: Build and maintain support networks with friends, family, or community groups. Support networks provide emotional support, practical assistance, and a sense of connection.

Regular Check-Ins

- Family Wellness Assessments: Energize family wellness by holding regular check-ins where you openly discuss each member's needs, goals, and concerns. Use these conversations to proactively tackle any issues, making dynamic adjustments to routines and practices that keep your family thriving.

- Celebrating Milestones: Turn family milestones into joyful celebrations! Recognize both individual and collective achievements with enthusiasm to foster a sense of accomplishment and create lasting memories. These celebrations not only boost motivation but also infuse your family life with positivity and excitement.

- Embracing Change: Embrace change with a spirit of adventure! Be ready to adapt family practices and routines as life evolves, transforming challenges into opportunities for growth. Flexibility and a willingness to adjust ensure that your family remains resilient and joyful through all of life's transitions.

- Continuous Improvement: Make continuous improvement an exhilarating journey! Stay curious and proactive in seeking new strategies to enhance family wellness. Learn from your experiences, experiment with innovative ideas, and celebrate the progress that elevates your family's well-being to new heights.

Chapter 8: Nurturing Growth and Development

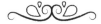

Nurturing a child's growth and development is one of the most fulfilling aspects of parenting. It involves providing the right environment, stimuli, and support to help a child reach their full potential. This chapter delves into various aspects of fostering growth, including stimulating cognitive development, supporting physical milestones, and encouraging emotional and social skills.

8.1 Stimulating Cognitive Development

Early Learning Opportunities

- Interactive Play: Engage your child in interactive play that challenges their thinking and problem-solving skills. Toys like building blocks, puzzles, and educational games can stimulate cognitive development by encouraging exploration and creativity.

- Reading Together: Establish a reading routine to enhance language skills and cognitive growth. Reading aloud to your child not only improves their vocabulary but also fosters a love for books and learning. Choose a variety of genres and themes to broaden their understanding and imagination.

- Curiosity and Exploration: Encourage curiosity by creating a stimulating environment that invites exploration. Provide safe spaces and opportunities for your child to investigate their interests, whether it's through nature walks, science experiments, or artistic activities.

Encouraging Critical Thinking

- Ask Open-Ended Questions: Promote critical thinking by asking open-ended questions that require more than a yes or no answer. Questions like "What do you think will happen if we mix these colors?" or "How do you think we could solve this problem?" encourage your child to think deeply and develop problem-solving skills.

- Support Independence: Allow your child to make choices and decisions within set boundaries. This practice fosters independence and critical thinking by giving them opportunities to weigh options and experience the consequences of their choices.

8.2 Supporting Physical Milestones

Promoting healthy growth involves providing a balanced diet, encouraging physical activity, and ensuring adequate rest. To support your child's physical development, offer a varied diet rich in essential nutrients, including fruits, vegetables, whole grains, and proteins, to deliver the necessary vitamins and minerals. Regular physical activity is crucial, so encourage activities such as running, jumping, climbing, and dancing, which help develop strength, coordination, and balance. Additionally, prioritize sufficient rest by establishing a consistent bedtime routine and creating a calming sleep environment to promote restful and restorative sleep.

Supporting Motor Skill Development

- Fine Motor Skills: Engage in activities that develop fine motor skills, such as drawing, writing, and manipulating small objects. These activities help improve hand-eye coordination and dexterity.

- Gross Motor Skills: Support the development of gross motor skills through activities that involve larger muscle groups, such as running, jumping, and playing sports. Outdoor play and active games are excellent ways to enhance these skills.

8.3 Encouraging Emotional and Social Skills

Building Emotional Intelligence

- Empathy and Understanding: Teach empathy by discussing emotions and modeling compassionate behavior. Encourage your child to recognize and understand their own feelings and those of others. Use real-life situations and stories to illustrate empathy and kindness.

- Emotional Regulation: Support your child in learning how to manage their emotions effectively. Teach techniques for calming down and coping with stress, such as deep breathing, mindfulness, and expressing feelings through words or creative outlets.

Developing Social Skills

- Positive Social Interactions: Facilitate opportunities for your child to interact with peers through play dates, group activities, and team sports. Positive social interactions help develop communication skills, cooperation, and friendship.

- Conflict Resolution: Teach your child conflict resolution skills by modeling and practicing problem-solving techniques. Encourage them to use "I" statements, listen actively, and work towards mutually agreeable solutions in disagreements.

8.4 Fostering Creativity and Imagination

Encouraging creative expression and nurturing a love for lifelong learning are integral to a child's development. To foster creativity, provide a variety of artistic materials such as crayons, paints, clay, and crafting supplies, and encourage activities like drawing, painting, crafting, and sculpting. For instance, you might set up a dedicated art station where your child can freely create their own masterpieces or work on themed craft projects. Engage in role-playing games, such as pretending to be characters from their favorite stories or creating new scenarios with toys, and storytelling sessions where they can invent their own tales. These activities stimulate imagination, enhance language skills, and build a sense of wonder.

Support creative exploration by exposing your child to diverse experiences. Plan visits to museums like a local children's museum or an art gallery, attend live performances such as theater shows or concerts, and explore nature through hiking or trips to botanical gardens. These experiences provide fresh ideas and perspectives. Celebrate and support their originality by encouraging them to pursue their passions, such as enrolling them in a dance class or a music lesson if they show interest. Offer opportunities for them to showcase their talents, such as participating in community art shows or school performances.

To nurture a love for lifelong learning, foster curiosity and exploration by supporting your child's interests with resources like educational books, science kits, or online courses related to their passions. Make learning enjoyable by incorporating educational elements into playtime. For example, use games like "Science Experiments at Home" kits, interactive geography puzzles, or math games to teach new concepts in a fun and engaging way. By combining these approaches, you help your child develop a rich, creative, and inquisitive mind that embraces learning and growth throughout their life.

Promoting a Growth Mindset

- Emphasizing Effort and Persistence: Encourage a growth mindset by praising effort and persistence rather than just outcomes. Help your child understand that learning and improvement come from practice and dedication.

- Embracing Challenges: Support your child in facing challenges and viewing them as opportunities for growth. Provide encouragement and guidance as they navigate difficulties and celebrate their progress and resilience.

Conclusion

Nurturing a child's growth and development requires a multi-faceted approach that integrates physical, emotional, cognitive, and creative aspects of their lives. By focusing on balanced nutrition, regular physical activity, and adequate rest, you lay the groundwork for healthy physical development. Encouraging creative expression through artistic activities and role-playing not only enhances imagination but also supports language development and emotional well-being.

Supporting creative exploration by exposing your child to diverse experiences and celebrating their unique talents fosters a sense of wonder and originality. Nurturing a love for lifelong learning involves nurturing curiosity and making educational activities engaging and enjoyable. By providing a stimulating environment that balances structured activities with opportunities for free exploration, you create a foundation for continuous growth and a lifelong enthusiasm for learning.

Incorporating these strategies into daily life helps build a well-rounded, resilient, and curious individual prepared to navigate the world's complexities with confidence and creativity. As we conclude this journey through holistic approaches to family wellness and motherhood, remember that each step you take in fostering your child's development enriches not only their lives but also strengthens the fabric of your family's shared experiences and growth. Your commitment to nurturing these aspects will lead to a vibrant, dynamic, and fulfilling family life where every member thrives and flourishes.

Please leave a review! Thank you for reading!

References

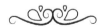

Books:

1. Armstrong, H. (2017). The Holistic Guide to Integrative Pediatrics: A Practical Approach to Children's Health. Springer.
2. Baker, M. (2021). Nurturing Your Child's Development: A Holistic Approach to Parenting. Harper Collins.
3. Cassidy, J., & Shaver, P. R. (2016).Handbook of Attachment: Theory, Research, and Clinical Applications. Guilford Press.
4. Friedman, M., & Mandel, D. (2018). The New Health Rules: Simple Changes to Achieve Whole-Body Wellness. Workman Publishing.
5. Kabat-Zinn, J. (2013). Wherever You Go, There You Are: Mindfulness Meditation in Everyday Life. Hyperion.

Research Articles:
6. Davis, E., & Carter, E. (2019). "The Impact of Holistic Interventions on Maternal and Infant Health: A Review of the Literature." Journal of Maternal and Child Health, 23(4),

456-467.

7. Johnson, S., & Miller, K. (2020). "Mindfulness-Based Stress Reduction for Parents: A Systematic Review." Pediatrics, 145(6), e20193448.

8. O'Connor, M., & Nock, M. K. (2021). "The Role of Nutrition in Child Development: A Holistic Perspective." *Nutrition Reviews, 79(2), 108-122.

Websites:

9. American Academy of Pediatrics (AAP). (2023). "Healthy-Children.org: Holistic Approaches to Child Health." Retrieved from https://www.healthychildren.org

10. National Center for Complementary and Integrative Health (NCCIH). (2024).** "Herbal Medicine." Retrieved from https://nccih.nih.gov/health/herbs

11. Mindful.org. (2024). "Mindfulness Practices for Families." Retrieved from https://www.mindful.orgOnline Resources:

12. WebMD. (2024). "Holistic Health: What Is It?" Retrieved from https://www.webmd.com/holistic-health

13. National Parenting Center. (2024). "Promoting Emotional and Social Development in Children." Retrieved from https://www.tnpc.com

All Natural Recipes

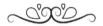

Ginger-Lemon Honey Tea

Ingredients:
- 1 fresh lemon
- 2-inch piece of fresh ginger root
- 1 tablespoon raw honey
- 2 cups water
- Optional: a few sprigs of fresh mint or a pinch of cayenne pepper

Instructions:

1. Prepare the Ginger:
- Peel the ginger root and slice it thinly. This helps to release more of its beneficial compounds.
2. Boil the Water:
- In a medium saucepan, bring 2 cups of water to a boil.
3. Add Ginger:

- Add the sliced ginger to the boiling water. Reduce the heat to low and let it simmer for about 10 minutes. This allows the ginger to infuse the water with its soothing properties.

4. Prepare the Lemon:
- While the ginger is simmering, cut the lemon in half. Squeeze the juice from one half into a mug, removing any seeds. You can slice the other half into wedges for garnish, if desired.

5. Strain the Tea:
- After the ginger has simmered, strain the tea into the mug with the lemon juice, discarding the ginger slices.

6. Add Honey:
- Stir in the raw honey until it dissolves completely. Honey has natural antimicrobial properties and adds a soothing sweetness.

7. Optional Additions:
- For an extra boost, add a few fresh mint leaves or a pinch of cayenne pepper. Mint can help clear nasal congestion, and cayenne pepper may provide additional relief from sore throat.

8. Enjoy:
- Sip the tea slowly while it's warm. It can be consumed several times a day to help ease cold symptoms and support your recovery.

Garlic-Honey Immunity Tonic

Ingredients:
- 5-6 cloves of fresh garlic
- 1/2 cup raw honey
- 1 tablespoon apple cider vinegar
- Juice of 1 lemon (optional)

Instructions:

1. Prepare the Garlic:
- Peel and finely chop or crush the garlic cloves. Crushing garlic releases allicin, a compound with potent antimicrobial properties.
2. Combine Ingredients:
- In a clean glass jar, add the finely chopped garlic.
3. Add Honey:
- Pour the raw honey over the garlic. Raw honey has natural antibacterial properties and acts as a preservative, helping to infuse the garlic's benefits.
4. Add Apple Cider Vinegar:
- Add the apple cider vinegar. This ingredient has antimicrobial properties and can help with digestion and immune support.

5. Optional Lemon Juice:
- If desired, add the juice of one lemon for extra vitamin C, which supports the immune system.
6. Mix and Infuse:
- Stir the mixture well to combine. Seal the jar and let it sit at room temperature for at least 24 hours to allow the flavors to meld and the garlic to infuse into the honey.
7. Store and Use:
- Store the jar in a cool, dark place. The tonic can be consumed by taking a teaspoon up to 3 times a day, especially when you feel a cold coming on or need an immune boost.
8. Enjoy:
- Take the tonic directly or mix it into warm water or herbal tea for easier consumption.

Super food Salad

Ingredients:
- For the Salad:
- 2 cups mixed greens (such as spinach, kale, and arugula)
- 1 cup cooked quinoa (cooled)
- 1/2 cup shredded red cabbage
- 1/2 cup cherry tomatoes, halved
- 1/2 avocado, diced
- 1/4 cup blueberries
- 1/4 cup walnuts, chopped
- 2 tablespoons pumpkin seeds
- 1/4 cup feta cheese or vegan cheese (optional)

- For the Dressing:
- 3 tablespoons extra-virgin olive oil
- 1 tablespoon apple cider vinegar
- 1 tablespoon lemon juice
- 1 teaspoon Dijon mustard
- 1 teaspoon honey or maple syrup
- 1 clove garlic, minced
- Salt and pepper to taste

Instructions:

1. Prepare the Ingredients:
   - If not already done, cook the quinoa according to package instructions and let it cool.
   - Wash and dry the mixed greens.
2. Assemble the Salad:
   - In a large salad bowl, combine the mixed greens, cooked

quinoa, shredded red cabbage, cherry tomatoes, avocado, blueberries, walnuts, and pumpkin seeds.

3. Make the Dressing:

- In a small bowl or jar, whisk together the olive oil, apple cider vinegar, lemon juice, Dijon mustard, honey or maple syrup, minced garlic, salt, and pepper until well combined.

4. Dress the Salad:

- Drizzle the dressing over the salad and toss gently to combine. Ensure all ingredients are evenly coated with the dressing.

5. Top and Serve:

- If using, sprinkle the feta or vegan cheese over the top of the salad.

- Serve immediately for the freshest flavor and texture.

Benefits:

- Mixed Greens: High in vitamins A, C, and K, and antioxidants.

- Quinoa: A complete protein with essential amino acids and fiber.

- Red Cabbage: Rich in vitamins C and K, and antioxidants.

- Avocado: Provides healthy fats and potassium.

- Blueberries: Packed with antioxidants and vitamins.

- Walnuts: Good source of omega-3 fatty acids and protein.

- Pumpkin Seeds: Rich in magnesium, iron, and zinc.

Blue Spirulina Superfood Smoothie

Ingredients:

- 1 banana (preferably frozen for a creamier texture)
- 1/2 cup Greek yogurt or a plant-based alternative (for added protein and creaminess)

- 1 cup fresh spinach or kale
- 1/2 cup blueberries (fresh or frozen)
- 1/2 cup pineapple chunks (fresh or frozen)
- 1 tablespoon blue spirulina powder
- 1 tablespoon chia seeds (for added fiber and omega-3s)
- 1 cup almond milk or your preferred plant-based milk (adjust for desired thickness)
- 1 teaspoon honey or maple syrup (optional, for extra sweetness)
- Ice cubes (optional, for a thicker consistency)

Instructions:

1. Prepare Ingredients:
- Peel and slice the banana. If you haven't done so already, wash the spinach or kale.
2. Blend the Smoothie:
- In a blender, combine the banana, Greek yogurt, spinach or kale, blueberries, pineapple chunks, blue spirulina powder, chia seeds, and almond milk.
- If you like your smoothie colder or thicker, add a few ice cubes.
3. Sweeten and Blend:
- Add honey or maple syrup if you prefer a sweeter smoothie. Blend on high until smooth and creamy. Adjust the consistency with more almond milk if needed.
4. Serve:
- Pour the smoothie into a glass and enjoy immediately for the best taste and texture.

Benefits:

- Blue Spirulina: Rich in protein, antioxidants, and essential nutrients like B vitamins and iron. It also has powerful anti-inflammatory and detoxifying properties.
- Banana: Provides natural sweetness, potassium, and dietary fiber.
- Greek Yogurt: Adds protein and probiotics for gut health.
- Spinach/Kale: Packed with vitamins A, C, K, and folate, and provides a dose of iron and antioxidants.
- Blueberries: High in antioxidants and vitamins C and K.
- Pineapple: Contains bromelain, which may aid digestion and reduce inflammation.
- Chia Seeds: A good source of omega-3 fatty acids, fiber, and protein.

Classic Sourdough Bread

Ingredients:

- For the Starter
    - 1 cup (120g) all-purpose flour or whole wheat flour
    - 1/2 cup (120ml) water (room temperature)
    - 1 tablespoon active sourdough starter (Make your own or get from a friend or a bakery)

- For the Dough:
    - 1 cup (240ml) water (room temperature)
    - 2 cups (240g) all-purpose flour
    - 1 cup (120g) whole wheat flour
    - 1 1/2 teaspoons salt
    - 1 tablespoon sugar or honey (optional, for a touch of

sweetness)
 - 1 cup (240ml) sourdough starter (active and bubbly)

Instructions:

1. Prepare the Starter:
 - If you're making your own starter, mix 1 cup of flour with 1/2 cup of water in a clean jar. Cover loosely and let sit at room temperature for 24 hours. Feed the starter daily with equal parts flour and water for about 5-7 days until it's bubbly and has a tangy smell. If you have an established starter, you can skip this step.

2. Feed the Starter (if needed):
 - Feed your starter with equal parts flour and water 8-12 hours before you plan to make your dough. It should be active and bubbly.

3. Mix the Dough:
 - In a large bowl, combine the water and 1 cup of active sourdough starter. Stir in the all-purpose flour, whole wheat flour, salt, and optional sugar or honey. Mix until a shaggy dough forms.
 4. Knead the Dough:
 - Turn the dough out onto a lightly floured surface and knead for about 10 minutes until smooth and elastic. Alternatively, you can use a stand mixer with a dough hook attachment on medium speed for about 8 minutes.
 5.First Rise:
 - Place the dough in a lightly oiled bowl, cover it with a damp cloth or plastic wrap, and let it rise at room temperature for

4-6 hours, or until doubled in size. The rise time can vary depending on the temperature and activity of your starter.

6. Shape the Dough:

- Gently deflate the dough and shape it into a round loaf or place it into a lightly floured banneton (proofing basket). For a round loaf, place it on a parchment-lined baking sheet or a preheated Dutch oven.

7. Second Rise:

- Cover the dough and let it rise again for 1-2 hours, or until it has nearly doubled in size. This is known as the second rise or proof.

8. Preheat the Oven:

- Preheat your oven to 450°F (230°C). If you're using a Dutch oven, place it inside the oven to preheat as well.

9. Score the Dough:

- Just before baking, use a sharp knife or razor blade to score the top of the loaf. This allows the bread to expand and helps control the shape of the crust.

10. Bake the Bread:

- If using a Dutch oven, carefully remove it from the oven, place the dough inside, and cover with the lid. Bake for 30 minutes, then remove the lid and bake for an additional 15-20 minutes, or until the loaf is deep brown and sounds hollow when tapped on the bottom.

- If baking on a baking sheet, bake for 35-40 minutes until the crust is golden brown and the loaf sounds hollow when tapped.

11. Cool the Bread:

- Allow the bread to cool completely on a wire rack before slicing. This ensures the interior is fully set and enhances the texture.

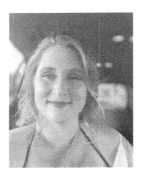

About the Author

Biography of Kate Rose

Kate is a devoted mother to two sons, David Jr. and Jordan, and a passionate advocate for holistic living. With a degree in Exercise Science and a career in personal training, Kate was already committed to health and wellness. However, a reformative experience during the delivery of her first son, David Jr., sparked a profound interest in holistic living beyond exercise and nutrition.

Driven by a desire to provide the best for her children, Kate delved into researching the impact of food, cleaning products, and environmental toxins on health. This journey led her to make significant lifestyle changes, focusing on creating a healthier and safer environment for her family.

Today, Kate continues to inspire others with her dedication to holistic living, blending her professional background with a personal commitment to well-being for herself and her family.